Herd Immunity For Infectious Diseases

(Advances in herd immunity)

Dr. Brian Chris

Chapter 1: Introduction to Infectious Disease

Infectious diseases are caused by harmful microorganisms invading the body, such as bacteria, viruses, fungi, and parasites. These pathogens can enter the body through various routes, including the respiratory tract, gastrointestinal tract, and through breaks in the skin. Once inside the body, they can replicate, thereby resulting to illness by disrupting normal cellular functions and triggering immune responses.

One of the key features of infectious diseases is their ability to be transmitted from person to person, either directly through close contact or indirectly through contaminated objects or surfaces. This transmission can occur through the air, water, food, or bodily fluids. Understanding the modes of transmission is critical for controlling the spread of infectious diseases and implementing effective prevention measures.

The impact of infectious diseases on a population can vary significantly depending on factors such as the pathogen's virulence, the host's immune response, and the environment in which the disease occurs. Some infectious diseases can cause mild symptoms and resolve on their own, while others can be severe, life-threatening, or lead to long-term complications. Vulnerable populations, such as the elderly, young children, and immunocompromised individuals, are at higher risk of developing severe forms of infectious diseases.

Preventing and controlling infectious diseases require a multi-faceted approach that includes vaccination, good hygiene practices, sanitation, outbreak surveillance, and prompt treatment of infected individuals. Vaccination is one of the most effective strategies for preventing infectious diseases by stimulating the immune system to produce protective antibodies against specific pathogens. Additionally, promoting good hygiene practices, such as handwashing, proper sanitation, and safe food handling, can help reduce the risk of infection and spread of diseases.

Infectious diseases pose a significant global health challenge, impacting populations worldwide and requiring coordinated efforts from healthcare providers, public health authorities, researchers, and policymakers to address effectively. Emerging infectious diseases, such as COVID-19, Ebola, and Zika virus, highlight the importance of preparedness, rapid response, and global collaboration in the face of new and evolving threats. Advancements in technology, such as genomics, bioinformatics, and big data analytics, have revolutionised our understanding of infectious diseases and improved our ability to detect, track, and respond to outbreaks in real-time.

In conclusion, infectious diseases remain a major public health concern with significant implications for global health security and wellbeing. Understanding the basic principles of infectious diseases, including their causes, transmission, prevention, and control, is essential for healthcare professionals, policymakers, and the general public to effectively combat these threats. By working together through interdisciplinary collaboration and innovation, we can strive to prevent, control, and ultimately eradicate infectious diseases for a healthier and safer future for all.

Chapter 2: Understanding Vaccines and Immunization

Vaccines are biological products known for helping the immune system develop resistance against specific diseases by creating an immune response similar to that produced by the natural infection itself. They typically contain weakened or inactivated parts of microbes, such as bacteria or viruses, or even just small pieces of them. When administered, vaccines prompt the immune system to create antibodies to fight off the infection. This way, the body's immune system learns to recognize and remember the pathogen, enabling it to react more effectively to future encounters with the actual disease-causing agent.

Immunization is the process through which a person becomes protected against a disease through vaccination. It is a critical component of public health, as it not only prevents individuals from getting sick but also helps in reducing the spread of infectious diseases within communities. By achieving high vaccination rates, a phenomenon known as herd immunity can be established, providing indirect protection to vulnerable populations such as individuals who cannot be vaccinated due to medical reasons or those with weakened immune systems.

One of the key benefits of vaccines is their ability to prevent the spread of infectious diseases. When a significant portion of a population is vaccinated, the transmission of the disease is hindered, leading to lower infection rates and ultimately protecting vulnerable individuals who are unable to get vaccinated. This concept is particularly important in preventing the outbreak of diseases like measles, polio, and influenza, where high vaccination coverage is crucial for effective disease control.

Vaccines undergo rigorous testing and assessment before being approved for public use to ensure their safety and effectiveness. Clinical trials are conducted to evaluate the vaccine's ability to provide protection against specific diseases while monitoring for any adverse effects. Continuous monitoring post-approval ensures that any potential safety concerns are promptly addressed, maintaining public confidence in vaccination programs. Furthermore, regulatory bodies oversee the production, distribution, and administration of vaccines to uphold quality standards and safety protocols.

Understanding the basics of vaccines and immunisation is essential for making informed decisions about one's health and well-being. Effective communication by healthcare professionals and public health authorities plays a crucial role in educating the public about the importance of vaccination in preventing disease outbreaks and protecting individuals and communities. Addressing misinformation and myths surrounding vaccines is key to promoting vaccine acceptance and uptake, ultimately contributing to improved public health outcomes.

While vaccines have been instrumental in controlling many deadly diseases, vaccine hesitancy remains a challenge in some communities. Factors such as misinformation, lack of access to healthcare, and distrust in the healthcare system can contribute to vaccine hesitancy. Efforts to address these barriers include improving access to vaccines, enhancing public education campaigns, and fostering trust in healthcare providers. By addressing these challenges, the overall success of immunization programs can be enhanced, leading to better health outcomes for all.

In conclusion, vaccines and immunization play a vital role in protecting individuals and communities from infectious diseases. By stimulating the body's immune response, vaccines help develop immunity to specific diseases, preventing their spread and reducing the burden on healthcare systems. Through rigorous testing, monitoring, and communication efforts, vaccines continue to be a cornerstone of public health initiatives worldwide. By understanding the science behind vaccines, addressing vaccine hesitancy, and ensuring equitable access to immunization, we can work together to build healthier and more resilient communities for the future.

Chapter 3: Concepts of Herd Immunity

Herd immunity, also known as community immunity, is a concept that describes a situation where a sufficient proportion of a population is immune to a particular infectious disease, either through vaccination or previous exposure, thereby providing indirect protection to those who are not immune. This concept is fundamental in public health as it helps control the spread of infectious diseases, especially in communities where vaccination rates are high. When a significant portion of the population is immune, the transmission of the disease slows down, making it less likely for the vulnerable individuals to come into contact with the infectious agent.

The threshold required to achieve herd immunity varies depending on the contagiousness of the disease. For highly contagious infections like measles, a vaccination rate of around 95% is typically needed to prevent outbreaks. However, for diseases with lower transmission rates, the herd immunity threshold may be lower. Understanding these thresholds is crucial for designing effective vaccination strategies and public health campaigns to protect populations from infectious diseases.Herd immunity not only protects individuals who cannot be vaccinated due to health conditions or age but also helps prevent the re-emergence of certain diseases that have been effectively controlled through vaccination programs. By reducing the overall prevalence of a disease in a population, herd immunity creates a buffer that limits the spread of infections and minimises the risk of outbreaks. This collective immunity is essential for protecting vulnerable populations, such as infants, elderly individuals, and individuals with compromised immune systems.However, achieving and maintaining herd immunity can be challenging, especially in the face of vaccine hesitancy, misinformation, and logistical barriers to vaccination. When vaccination rates drop below the threshold necessary for herd immunity, the risk of outbreaks increases, leading to a resurgence of preventable diseases. To address this issue, public health efforts focus on improving vaccination coverage, promoting vaccine confidence, and debunking myths surrounding vaccines to ensure the health and safety of communities.The COVID-19 pandemic has brought renewed attention to the concept of herd immunity, as achieving widespread immunity through vaccination has been identified as a crucial step in controlling the spread of the virus. With the development and deployment of COVID-19 vaccines, governments and health organisations worldwide are working to increase vaccination rates to reach herd immunity levels and minimise the impact of the pandemic. Public health interventions, such as mass vaccination campaigns and education initiatives, play a vital role in achieving herd immunity and protecting populations from the devastating effects of infectious diseases.In conclusion, herd immunity is a powerful public health concept that plays a critical role in protecting populations from infectious diseases. By establishing a level of immunity within a community, herd immunity reduces the risk of disease transmission and safeguards vulnerable individuals who are unable to be vaccinated. Understanding the principles of herd immunity is essential for designing effective vaccination strategies, promoting public health initiatives, and preventing outbreaks of contagious diseases. Through collective efforts to increase vaccination coverage and promote vaccine confidence, communities can achieve and maintain herd immunity, ensuring the health and well-being of society as a whole.

Chapter 4: History of Herd Immunity and Its Impact on Public Health

Herd immunity, also known as community immunity, is a concept that has been crucial in the history of public health throughout the ages. The idea behind herd immunity is that when a significant portion of a population becomes immune to a particular infectious disease, either through vaccination or previous exposure, the spread of the disease is significantly reduced. This indirect protection benefits those who are not immune, such as those who are too young or too ill to be vaccinated. The concept of herd immunity dates back to the early 20th century when it was first proposed by researchers to explain the decline in infectious disease outbreaks after a certain percentage of the population became immune.

One of the earliest examples of herd immunity in practice can be seen in the case of smallpox. Smallpox was a devastating disease that caused widespread death and suffering throughout history. In the 18th century, the practice of variolation, a precursor to vaccination, was used in some cultures to induce immunity to smallpox. As more people became immune through variolation or natural infection, the overall prevalence of the disease decreased, leading to a form of herd immunity that contributed to the eventual eradication of smallpox.

The impact of herd immunity on public health cannot be overstated. By reducing the spread of infectious diseases within a population, herd immunity plays a critical role in protecting vulnerable individuals who may be unable to be vaccinated. This includes infants, elderly people, and individuals with weakened immune systems. Herd immunity is especially important for preventing outbreaks of highly contagious diseases such as measles, mumps, and whooping cough, which can spread rapidly in communities with low vaccination rates.

The introduction of vaccines has been a game-changer in the history of herd immunity and public health. Vaccination programs have been instrumental in achieving and maintaining high levels of immunity within populations, leading to the control or eradication of many infectious diseases. For example, the widespread use of the measles vaccine has contributed to a significant reduction in measles cases and related deaths globally. Vaccines not only protect individuals who receive them but also contribute to the overall immunity of the community, thereby supporting herd immunity.

Despite the benefits of herd immunity, maintaining high vaccination coverage rates can be challenging due to various factors such as vaccine hesitancy, access issues, and misinformation. When vaccination rates dip below the threshold required for herd immunity, there is an increased risk of disease outbreaks and a potential loss of protection for vulnerable individuals. Recent outbreaks of measles in some regions have underscored the importance of promoting vaccine uptake and addressing barriers to vaccination to ensure herd immunity remains effective in protecting public health.

In recent years, the concept of herd immunity has garnered increased attention due to debates surrounding mandatory vaccination policies and the spread of misinformation about vaccines. Achieving and sustaining herd immunity requires a collective effort from individuals, healthcare professionals, policymakers, and public health authorities. Education, outreach programs, and initiatives to address vaccine hesitancy are essential components of maintaining high vaccination rates and protecting public health through herd immunity.

Looking ahead, the ongoing COVID-19 pandemic has highlighted the critical role of herd immunity in controlling the spread of infectious diseases. With the development and distribution of COVID-19 vaccines, there is hope that achieving herd immunity against the virus can bring an end to the pandemic and protect vulnerable populations. However, challenges such as vaccine distribution, vaccine acceptance, and the emergence of new variants underscore the need for a coordinated and comprehensive approach to vaccination efforts to reach sufficient levels of immunity within communities.

In conclusion, the history of herd immunity and its impact on public health demonstrate the importance of vaccination and collective immunity in preventing the spread of infectious diseases and protecting vulnerable populations. Through vaccination programs, public health initiatives, and community engagement, maintaining high levels of immunity within populations can help safeguard individuals who are most at risk. Understanding the history and significance of herd immunity can inform current efforts to promote vaccination, combat vaccine-preventable diseases, and ensure a healthier future for communities worldwide.

Chapter 5: Mathematical Models of Herd Immunity

Herd immunity, a concept rooted in mathematical modelling, plays a crucial role in understanding the dynamics of infectious diseases within populations. By employing mathematical models, scientists and public health experts can predict how diseases spread and determine the optimal strategies for controlling them. One key aspect of herd immunity is that it describes the level of immunity in a population that is necessary to prevent sustained transmission of a disease. Mathematical models of herd immunity consider factors such as the transmissibility of the disease, the effectiveness of vaccines, and the structure of the population to estimate the threshold for achieving herd immunity.

Mathematical models of herd immunity often incorporate epidemiological parameters such as the basic reproduction number (R0), which represents the average number of secondary infections generated from one infected individual in a completely susceptible population. These models can help determine the proportion of individuals that need to be immune to prevent an outbreak, known as the herd immunity threshold. By adjusting various parameters in the model, researchers can explore different scenarios and interventions to achieve herd immunity and control the spread of infectious diseases.

One common type of mathematical model used to simulate herd immunity is the compartmental model, which divides the population into compartments based on their disease status (e.g., susceptible, infected, recovered) and tracks the flow of individuals between these compartments over time. These models can provide insights into how vaccination campaigns, natural immunity, and other public health measures impact the spread of diseases and the level of immunity within a population. By running simulations with different assumptions and inputs, researchers can assess the effectiveness of various strategies for achieving and maintaining herd immunity.

Another important aspect of mathematical models of herd immunity is their ability to account for complex interactions within populations, such as age structure, spatial dynamics, and individual behaviours. By incorporating these factors into the models, researchers can better understand how different populations may require tailored approaches to achieving herd immunity. For example, populations with high levels of mixing among individuals may require higher vaccination coverage to reach the herd immunity threshold compared to populations with lower levels of interaction.

Mathematical models of herd immunity are also instrumental in guiding public health policies and vaccination strategies. These models can inform decisions on vaccine allocation, timing of interventions, and monitoring of infectious diseases within populations. By combining mathematical modelling with empirical data and epidemiological studies, public health officials can develop evidence-based strategies to maximise the benefits of herd immunity while minimising the risks of disease outbreaks. Overall, mathematical models of herd immunity serve as powerful tools for understanding the dynamics of infectious diseases and designing effective interventions to protect populations from the threat of outbreaks.

Chapter 6: Vaccine Development and Distribution Strategies

Vaccine development and distribution strategies play a crucial role in protecting populations from infectious diseases and pandemics. The process of developing a vaccine involves rigorous scientific research and testing to ensure safety and efficacy. Scientists typically follow a series of steps that include preclinical studies, clinical trials in human subjects, regulatory approval, and post-marketing surveillance. These stages are essential for assessing the vaccine's safety, effectiveness, and potential side effects before widespread distribution.

Once a vaccine passes through the development phase, the challenge shifts to distribution strategies to ensure wide accessibility and coverage. Vaccine distribution involves a complex supply chain that includes production, storage, transportation, and delivery to vaccination centers. To streamline this process, countries and organizations often work together to establish distribution networks that can reach remote or underserved populations efficiently.

Strategies for vaccine distribution also involve prioritizing target populations based on risk factors such as age, occupation, health status, and geographic location. In the case of pandemics or outbreaks, frontline healthcare workers, elderly individuals, and individuals with underlying health conditions are typically given priority access to vaccines. This approach helps to contain the spread of the disease and protect those most at risk of severe illness or complications.

Efforts to develop and distribute vaccines are often supported by public health agencies, governments, pharmaceutical companies, and non-profit organizations. Collaboration between these stakeholders is crucial for ensuring timely access to vaccines, especially in emergencies. Additionally, funding, infrastructure, and partnerships play a significant role in accelerating the development and deployment of vaccines to address global health challenges.

In recent years, technological advancements have transformed vaccine development and distribution processes. Innovations such as mRNA vaccines have shown great promise in rapidly developing effective vaccines against emerging pathogens like SARS-CoV-2. Furthermore, digital technologies, real-time data tracking, and artificial intelligence are being leveraged to enhance the efficiency of vaccine distribution and monitoring of vaccination coverage.

To address issues of vaccine hesitancy and misinformation, communication and education campaigns are essential components of effective distribution strategies. Providing accurate information about vaccines, addressing concerns about safety and efficacy, and promoting trust in the healthcare system are key to increasing vaccine acceptance and coverage. Community engagement, partnerships with local leaders, and culturally sensitive messaging can help improve vaccine uptake rates and public health outcomes.

In conclusion, vaccine development and distribution strategies are vital components of public health systems worldwide. By investing in research, manufacturing, and efficient distribution networks, countries can strengthen their preparedness for future health threats and pandemics. Collaboration, innovation, and equitable access to vaccines are key principles that guide efforts to protect populations from infectious diseases and improve global health outcomes. As technology continues to advance, it is important to adapt strategies to meet evolving challenges and ensure that vaccines reach those who need them most.

Chapter 7: Challenges in Achieving Herd Immunity

One of the critical challenges in achieving herd immunity is vaccine hesitancy. This reluctance or refusal to vaccinate stems from various factors, including misinformation, lack of trust in the healthcare system, and concerns about vaccine safety. As a result, reaching the high vaccination rates necessary for herd immunity becomes increasingly difficult when a significant portion of the population is hesitant or resistant to getting vaccinated.

Another challenge is the uneven distribution of vaccines globally. While some wealthier countries have secured ample vaccine supplies and made significant progress in vaccinating their populations, many low- and middle-income countries struggle to access an adequate supply of vaccines. This inequality hinders efforts to achieve herd immunity on a global scale, as the virus can continue to spread and mutate in areas with lower vaccination rates.

 Variants of the virus present a significant challenge to achieving herd immunity. As the virus mutates, new variants with potentially increased transmissibility or resistance to existing vaccines can emerge. These variants can hinder efforts to achieve herd immunity by potentially evading immunity acquired through vaccination or natural infection, requiring updated vaccines or additional booster doses to maintain protection.

Compliance with public health measures and guidelines is essential for achieving herd immunity, but challenges arise when individuals or communities do not adhere to these measures consistently. Factors like pandemic fatigue, misinformation, or complacency can lead to lapses in behaviour that contribute to ongoing transmission of the virus, making it harder to reach the level of immunity needed to stop the spread effectively.

The duration of immunity provided by vaccines or natural infection is another challenge in achieving herd immunity. Uncertainties remain about how long immunity lasts after vaccination or infection, and whether individuals are at risk of reinfection over time. If immunity wanes or if new variants emerge that reduce vaccine effectiveness, achieving and maintaining herd immunity may require ongoing efforts to boost immunity through additional doses or updated vaccines.

Access barriers to vaccination, such as lack of transportation, limited availability of vaccination sites, or issues with vaccine affordability, can impede efforts to achieve herd immunity. In marginalised or underserved communities, these access barriers can widen existing disparities in vaccination rates, making it harder to reach the levels of immunity necessary to protect the entire population. and disinformation circulating online and in communities present a significant challenge to achieving herd immunity. False or misleading information about vaccines, their safety, and effectiveness can erode public trust in vaccination efforts and dissuade individuals from getting vaccinated. Countering misinformation and promoting accurate information are critical for building trust and increasing vaccine acceptance to achieve herd immunity.

Finally, the interconnected nature of our global society poses challenges to achieving herd immunity. Travel and trade across borders can facilitate the spread of the virus between countries, making it challenging to contain outbreaks and achieve widespread immunity on a global scale. Collaborative efforts and international cooperation are essential to address these challenges and work towards achieving herd immunity to bring the pandemic under control.

Chapter 8: Ethical Considerations in Herd Immunity Programs

Herd immunity programs, which aim to achieve a level of immunity within a population to prevent the spread of infectious diseases, raise significant ethical considerations. One key ethical consideration is the potential impact on vulnerable populations, such as individuals who cannot receive vaccinations due to medical reasons or those who are immune-compromised. It is essential to ensure that herd immunity programs do not inadvertently disproportionately harm these communities by leaving them at increased risk of infection. Strategies must be implemented to protect and support these vulnerable groups to prevent further health disparities.

Another ethical consideration in herd immunity programs is the issue of informed consent. Individuals should have access to accurate information about the risks and benefits of vaccines to make informed decisions about vaccination. It is vital that public health communication efforts prioritize transparency and provide clear, accessible information to promote informed consent. Respecting individuals' autonomy and ensuring that they have the necessary information to make decisions that align with their values and beliefs are essential ethical principles in herd immunity programs.

Furthermore, equity and justice are critical ethical considerations in herd immunity programs. It is crucial to ensure equitable access to vaccinations for all members of society, regardless of socio-economic status, race, ethnicity, or other factors. Efforts should be made to address barriers to vaccination, such as cost, transportation, language, or cultural factors, to promote equal opportunities for protection against infectious diseases. Failure to address these disparities can perpetuate existing health inequities and widen the gap between different populations.

The principle of beneficence is fundamental in the ethical framework of herd immunity programs. Policymakers and public health authorities have a duty to promote the well-being of the population by implementing effective vaccination strategies that prioritize the greater good. Balancing individual rights with the collective benefit of achieving herd immunity requires careful consideration of the potential risks and benefits of vaccination programs. Decision-makers must weigh the benefits of protecting the community against the potential harms of mandatory vaccination policies that may infringe on individual liberties.

Additionally, transparency and accountability are essential ethical considerations in herd immunity programs. Public health authorities should be transparent about the scientific evidence supporting vaccination recommendations and openly communicate any uncertainties or risks associated with vaccines. Building trust with the public through open dialogue and accountability mechanisms is crucial for the success of vaccination programs. It is essential to address public concerns, engage with communities, and involve stakeholders in the decision-making process to ensure that herd immunity programs uphold ethical standards and meet the needs of the population.

Moreover, balancing individual rights with societal obligations is a complex ethical challenge in herd immunity programs. While individuals have the right to make informed decisions about their health, their choices can impact the health and well-being of others in the community. This ethical dilemma raises questions about the limits of individual autonomy in the context of public health interventions. Respecting individual freedoms while promoting the common good requires finding a delicate balance that safeguards both personal liberty and collective well-being in herd immunity programs.

Another important ethical consideration in herd immunity programs is the principle of non-maleficence, which emphasizes the obligation to minimize harm and avoid unnecessary risks to individuals. While vaccines are generally considered safe and effective, there are potential risks associated with vaccination, such as adverse reactions or rare side effects. Public health authorities must carefully weigh the risks and benefits of vaccination programs to ensure that the benefits of achieving herd immunity outweigh any potential harms. Monitoring and evaluating the safety of vaccines and responding promptly to concerns are essential to maintaining public trust and confidence in vaccination programs.

In conclusion, ethical considerations play a crucial role in guiding the development and implementation of herd immunity programs. Upholding principles such as respect for individual autonomy, equity, justice, beneficence, transparency, and accountability is essential to ensure that vaccination efforts prioritize the well-being of the population while respecting individual rights and values. By addressing these ethical considerations thoughtfully and responsibly, public health authorities can foster trust, promote social cohesion, and effectively combat infectious diseases through herd immunity programs that prioritize the

health and welfare of all members of society.

Chapter 9: Communicating Science for Public Understanding

Communicating science to the general public is crucial in fostering public understanding and appreciation of scientific advancements. The public plays a key role in determining the societal impact of scientific research and findings. Effective communication helps bridge the gap between the scientific community and the public, facilitating informed decision-making and policy formation on issues that have scientific implications.

One of the challenges in communicating science to the public is the complexity of scientific concepts, which can be overwhelming for non-experts. Scientists and communicators need to employ clear and concise language, avoid jargon, and use relatable examples to make the information comprehensible to a broad audience. By simplifying complex topics without oversimplifying them, the public can better grasp the significance of scientific research and its relevance to their everyday lives.Visual aids, such as infographics, videos, and interactive tools, are instrumental in engaging the public and simplifying complex scientific information. These tools can help break down intricate concepts into digestible pieces, making them more accessible and compelling for a wider audience. By incorporating visuals alongside written content, communicators can enhance the effectiveness of their messages and capture the attention of diverse individuals.

Building trust is another vital aspect of communicating science for public understanding. Transparency, honesty, and accountability are essential for establishing credibility with the public. By openly sharing the methodology, data, and limitations of scientific studies, researchers can foster trust and confidence in their findings, encouraging the public to view scientific information as reliable and valuable.

Engaging with the public through various platforms, such as social media, public talks, workshops, and citizen science projects, can expand the reach of scientific communication and promote interactive learning experiences. By creating opportunities for dialogue and participation, scientists can address misconceptions, answer questions, and solicit feedback from the public, fostering a two-way exchange of knowledge and ideas.

Contextualising scientific information within real-world scenarios and addressing its implications for society can help the public connect with scientific content on a personal level. By highlighting the practical applications and potential risks of scientific advancements, communicators can demonstrate the relevance of science to pressing issues, such as health, environment, and technology, that impact individuals and communities.

Recognizing the diversity of perspectives, backgrounds, and interests within the public is essential for effective science communication. Tailoring messages to different audiences, considering cultural sensitivities, and acknowledging varying levels of prior knowledge can enhance the inclusivity and accessibility of scientific information. By adopting an audience-centered approach, communicators can better engage diverse individuals and foster a more inclusive understanding of science.

In conclusion, communicating science for public understanding requires clarity, engagement, trust, and inclusivity to bridge the gap between the scientific community and the general public. By employing effective communication strategies, utilising visual aids, building trust through transparency, engaging with the public, contextualising scientific information, and recognizing audience diversity, scientists and communicators can enhance public understanding of science and its impact on society. By promoting informed decision-making, critical thinking, and appreciation for science, effective communication efforts can empower the public to actively participate in discussions and debates on scientific issues that shape our world.

Chapter 10: Global Perspectives on Herd Immunity

Herd immunity is a concept that has gained significant attention and debate on a global scale, especially in the context of the COVID-19 pandemic. The concept refers to a situation where a sufficient portion of a population is immune to a specific infectious disease, either through vaccination or prior infection, thus providing indirect protection to those who are not immune. The percentage needed for herd immunity varies depending on the contagiousness of the particular disease, with estimates typically ranging from 60% to 90%.

On a global level, differing perspectives on herd immunity have emerged, reflecting a complex interplay of scientific understanding, public health strategies, and societal attitudes. Some countries have pursued herd immunity as a primary strategy to combat the pandemic, while others have prioritised measures like widespread vaccination campaigns and public health restrictions to control the spread of the virus. These divergent approaches have led to varying outcomes in terms of infection rates, healthcare system capacity, and economic impact.

In some regions, scepticism and mistrust towards vaccines have hindered efforts to achieve herd immunity. Misinformation, vaccine hesitancy, and cultural beliefs can all affect vaccination rates and the overall effectiveness of population immunity. Addressing these challenges requires a multifaceted approach involving public education, community engagement, and targeted interventions to build trust and increase vaccination uptake.

From a global health perspective, achieving herd immunity against diseases like COVID-19 is seen as a critical milestone in controlling and eventually halting the spread of the virus. However, disparities in vaccine access, distribution, and uptake pose significant challenges to realising this goal. International cooperation and solidarity are essential in ensuring equitable access to vaccines and supporting countries with limited resources to strengthen their vaccination programs.

The concept of herd immunity is not without its ethical considerations, particularly regarding issues of individual rights, public health mandates, and vaccine equity. Balancing the collective good with individual autonomy is a complex dilemma that policymakers, public health authorities, and communities must navigate in the pursuit of population immunity. Approaches that respect individual rights while prioritising public health goals are crucial for fostering trust and cooperation in efforts to achieve herd immunity.

Global perspectives on herd immunity also highlight the interconnected nature of health outcomes across borders. In an increasingly interconnected world, the success of achieving herd immunity in one country can have ripple effects on others through travel, trade, and migration. This underscores the importance of international collaboration in managing and controlling infectious diseases, highlighting the need for a coordinated, evidence-based approach to achieving herd immunity on a global scale.

As the world continues to grapple with the COVID-19 pandemic and other infectious disease threats, the concept of herd immunity remains a key focal point in discussions around public health strategies and disease control. Understanding the varying perspectives, challenges, and opportunities related to achieving population immunity can inform more effective and sustainable approaches to safeguarding global health and well-being. By fostering collaboration, innovation, and inclusivity, countries can work together towards a shared goal of achieving herd immunity and mitigating the impact of infectious diseases on a global scale.

Chapter 11: Case Studies of Successful Herd Immunity Campaigns

One notable case study of a successful herd immunity campaign can be seen in the small town of Temecula, California. Through a combination of targeted vaccination drives, community education programs, and widespread outreach efforts, the town was able to achieve a vaccination rate of over 95% among its residents. This high level of immunisation effectively created a protective barrier around vulnerable individuals who were unable to get vaccinated due to medical reasons, thereby significantly reducing the risk of outbreaks of diseases like measles or pertussis.

Another compelling example of a successful herd immunity campaign is found in the country of Rwanda. Facing a significant burden of preventable diseases, the Rwandan government launched a comprehensive vaccination program that aimed to reach every corner of the country. Through the use of mobile clinics, community health workers, and strong partnerships with international organisations, Rwanda managed to achieve one of the highest vaccination rates in Africa. As a result, the country saw a dramatic decrease in the prevalence of diseases like polio and measles, showcasing the power of herd immunity in protecting public health.

In the city of Stockholm, Sweden, a successful herd immunity campaign was carried out in response to a measles outbreak in 2017. The public health authorities swiftly organised mass vaccination clinics, implemented targeted outreach campaigns in affected communities, and worked closely with schools and childcare centres to ensure high vaccination coverage. As a result of these efforts, the outbreak was quickly contained, and the city was able to achieve herd immunity against measles, preventing further spread of the disease and safeguarding vulnerable populations.

The island nation of Maldives provides another compelling case study of a successful herd immunity campaign. Faced with a high incidence of vaccine-preventable diseases and a dispersed population across numerous atolls, the Maldivian government launched an extensive immunisation program that involved setting up vaccination centres in remote areas, training local health workers, and engaging with community leaders to promote vaccination. Through these efforts, the country was able to achieve high vaccination coverage rates, leading to a significant reduction in the incidence of diseases like rubella and diphtheria.

In the aftermath of the 2014-2016 Ebola outbreak in West Africa, the region witnessed a successful herd immunity campaign in Sierra Leone. Recognizing the importance of vaccination in preventing future outbreaks, the Sierra Leonean government collaborated with international partners to strengthen its immunisation program. By improving vaccine access, increasing community engagement, and building trust in healthcare systems, Sierra Leone was able to boost vaccination rates and create a protective shield against infectious diseases, showcasing the critical role of herd immunity in outbreak prevention.

On the other side of the globe, in the rural villages of Bhutan, a successful herd immunity campaign was carried out to combat the spread of hepatitis B. By leveraging the country's extensive network of healthcare workers, implementing door-to-door vaccination campaigns, and integrating vaccination services with routine healthcare visits, Bhutan was able to achieve high vaccination coverage rates across its population. This proactive approach not only led to a significant decline in the incidence of hepatitis B but also demonstrated the effectiveness of community-based strategies in achieving herd immunity.

In the urban slums of Mumbai, India, a compelling case study of a successful herd immunity campaign unfolded in response to a spike in cases of tuberculosis. Recognizing the importance of vaccination as a preventive measure, local health authorities partnered with community organisations, religious leaders, and NGOs to implement a targeted vaccination drive in high-risk areas. Through these collaborative efforts, Mumbai was able to improve vaccination coverage rates, reduce the transmission of tuberculosis, and protect vulnerable populations from the disease, underscoring the impact of herd immunity in combating infectious diseases.

Lastly, the campaign to eradicate smallpox serves as a historic example of a successful global herd immunity effort. Through an unprecedented global vaccination campaign led by the World Health Organization, smallpox was successfully eradicated in 1980, marking a monumental achievement in public health. By ensuring widespread vaccination coverage across continents, mobilising resources, and coordinating international cooperation, the world was able to eliminate smallpox and demonstrate the power of collective immunity in eradicating a deadly disease, setting a powerful precedent for future immunisation efforts against infectious diseases.

Chapter 12: Emerging Infectious Diseases and Herd Immunity

Emerging infectious diseases pose significant threats to global public health due to their unpredictable nature and potential for rapid spread. Factors such as increased global travel, urbanisation, and environmental changes have facilitated the emergence of new infectious diseases that can easily jump from animals to humans. These zoonotic diseases, like COVID-19, SARS, MERS, and Ebola, highlight the interconnectedness of human and animal health and the need for a coordinated response to control their spread. As these diseases emerge and evolve, understanding the concept of herd immunity becomes crucial in mitigating their impact on populations.

Herd immunity, also known as community immunity, is a form of indirect protection from infectious diseases that occurs when a significant proportion of a population becomes immune to the pathogen, either through vaccination or previous exposure. When enough individuals are immune, the spread of the infectious agent within the community is hindered, resulting in protection for those who are susceptible, such as individuals who cannot be vaccinated due to medical reasons. Herd immunity acts as a shield, reducing the overall burden of disease and preventing outbreaks from reaching vulnerable individuals.

Achieving herd immunity in a population can significantly reduce the transmission of infectious diseases, thereby providing protection to those who are unable to receive vaccinations or have weakened immune systems. For highly contagious diseases like measles, which require a high level of immunity to prevent outbreaks, a vaccination coverage rate of around 93-95% is necessary to establish herd immunity. However, the threshold for herd immunity varies depending on the infectious agent's characteristics, such as its contagiousness and the duration of immunity conferred by vaccination or natural infection.

While herd immunity is a powerful tool in controlling the spread of infectious diseases, its effectiveness can be compromised by various factors, including vaccine hesitancy, lack of access to vaccines, waning immunity over time, and the emergence of new variants that may evade immune responses. In the context of emerging infectious diseases, such as novel coronaviruses or influenza strains with pandemic potential, achieving herd immunity can be particularly challenging due to the lack of pre-existing immunity in the population and the rapid spread of the pathogen. In these cases, a multi-faceted approach that combines vaccination, public health measures, and surveillance is essential to prevent large-scale outbreaks.

The COVID-19 pandemic has underscored the importance of herd immunity in controlling the spread of the virus and reducing its impact on communities worldwide. Vaccination campaigns have played a central role in building immunity against SARS-CoV-2 and slowing transmission rates, leading to a decline in cases and hospitalizations in many regions. However, achieving herd immunity against COVID-19 has proven to be a complex task, with challenges such as vaccine inequity, misinformation, and complacency hindering vaccination efforts in some populations. As new variants continue to emerge, maintaining high vaccination coverage and strengthening public health infrastructure are critical to sustaining herd immunity and preventing future waves of infection.

In the context of emerging infectious diseases, global cooperation and coordination are essential to address the interconnected challenges posed by these pathogens. By sharing information, resources, and expertise, countries can work together to monitor and respond to emerging threats, enhance surveillance systems, and develop strategies for achieving and maintaining herd immunity on a global scale. Investments in research and development, vaccine distribution, and public health infrastructure are crucial to building resilience against future pandemics and ensuring that populations are better prepared to respond to emerging infectious diseases. By advancing our understanding of herd immunity and its role in disease control, we can strengthen our defences against emerging infectious threats and protect the health and well-being of individuals and communities worldwide.

Chapter 13: Technology and Innovations in Herd Immunity Strategies

Herd immunity is a critical concept in public health that helps protect entire populations from contagious diseases by ensuring a significant portion of individuals are immune. Technological advancements and innovations have played a crucial role in enhancing herd immunity strategies. From the development of vaccines to sophisticated tracking systems, technology has revolutionised the way we approach and achieve herd immunity, especially in the face of recent global health challenges.

One of the most significant technological advancements in herd immunity strategies is the development of vaccines. Vaccines have been instrumental in preventing the spread of infectious diseases by stimulating the immune system to produce antibodies without causing the disease itself. Rapid advancements in vaccine technology, such as mRNA vaccines, have revolutionised the field, leading to the development of highly effective vaccines against previously challenging diseases.

Digital Health Platforms

Digital health platforms have become indispensable tools in herd immunity strategies. These platforms leverage technology to streamline immunisation campaigns, track vaccination coverage, and monitor disease outbreaks in real-time. By collecting and analysing vast amounts of data, digital health platforms enable public health authorities to make informed decisions and quickly respond to emerging health threats, ultimately contributing to the achievement of herd immunity.

Telemedicine and Remote Monitoring**

Telemedicine and remote monitoring technologies have expanded access to healthcare services, particularly in underserved communities, enhancing vaccination efforts and overall herd immunity. These technologies allow healthcare providers to remotely assess patients, deliver virtual consultations, and monitor vaccine effectiveness, enabling timely interventions and follow-ups to ensure optimal immunisation coverage within populations.

Genomic Sequencing

Advancements in genomic sequencing technologies have revolutionised our understanding of infectious diseases and their transmission dynamics, significantly impacting herd immunity strategies. By sequencing the genomes of pathogens, researchers can track the evolution of diseases, identify potential vaccine targets, and monitor the spread of resistant strains, informing targeted vaccination campaigns and containment measures.

Artificial Intelligence and Machine Learning**

Artificial intelligence (AI) and machine learning algorithms are increasingly being utilised in herd immunity strategies to optimise vaccine distribution, predict disease trends, and identify high-risk populations. These technologies can analyse complex data sets, model various vaccination scenarios, and provide insights that help public health authorities allocate resources more efficiently and effectively to achieve herd immunity goals.

Wearable Devices and Health Tracking Apps**

Wearable devices and health tracking apps have empowered individuals to actively participate in herd immunity efforts by monitoring their health status, tracking vaccination schedules, and receiving alerts about potential exposure to infectious diseases. These technologies promote individual accountability and compliance with vaccination programs, contributing to overall community immunity and reducing the risk of disease transmission.

Collaborative Platforms and Data Sharing

Technology has facilitated global collaboration among health organisations, researchers, and policymakers to develop coordinated herd immunity strategies on a large scale. Collaborative platforms and data-sharing initiatives enable the rapid dissemination of critical information, best practices, and research findings, fostering a collective effort to achieve and sustain herd immunity against a wide range of infectious diseases worldwide. By leveraging technology and fostering partnerships, we can continue to innovate and improve herd immunity strategies for the benefit of public health and well-being.

Chapter 14: Future Trends and Opportunities in Herd Immunity

Enhanced vaccination technologies are likely to play a significant role in shaping the future of herd immunity. Advancements in vaccine development, such as the use of mRNA technology, are paving the way for more effective and rapid response to emerging infectious diseases. This holds promise for achieving herd immunity faster and more efficiently against a wide range of pathogens. Furthermore, the development of novel delivery systems like microneedle patches and oral vaccines could help overcome barriers to vaccination adoption, ultimately improving population-level immunity.

Digital health technologies are poised to revolutionise the way herd immunity is monitored and managed in the future. The integration of big data analytics, artificial intelligence, and digital surveillance tools can provide real-time insights into vaccination coverage, disease spread, and immunity levels within communities. By leveraging these technologies, public health officials can make informed decisions to target interventions, optimize vaccine distribution, and track progress towards achieving herd immunity goals.

Social media and online platforms have emerged as powerful tools for disseminating information and encouraging vaccine uptake among the public. Influencers, healthcare professionals, and grassroots organisations can leverage these channels to raise awareness about the importance of herd immunity, debunk misinformation, and promote vaccination campaigns. By harnessing the reach and engagement of social media, stakeholders can foster a culture of vaccination acceptance and collective responsibility towards achieving community immunity.

The concept of localised immunity hubs or "vaccine bubbles" may gain traction in the future as a strategy to bolster herd immunity within specific populations or settings. By promoting high vaccination coverage and immunity clustering in key community hubs such as schools, workplaces, or social gatherings, it is possible to create pockets of protection against infectious diseases. This targeted approach can help shield vulnerable groups and prevent outbreaks from spreading within interconnected networks.

Global collaborations and partnerships will be essential for addressing disparities in vaccination access and coverage, particularly in underserved regions or marginalised populations. Initiatives like COVAX have demonstrated the importance of equitable vaccine distribution to achieve herd immunity on a global scale. Continued investments in capacity building, technology transfer, and supply chain infrastructure are vital to ensuring that no community is left behind in the quest for widespread immunity.

The emergence of novel vaccine platforms, such as multi-epitope peptide vaccines and self-amplifying RNA vaccines, could offer new avenues for enhancing herd immunity against evolving pathogens. These next-generation vaccines have the potential to confer broader protection, stimulate robust immune responses, and overcome challenges related to virus mutation and immune evasion. By diversifying the vaccine portfolio and leveraging cutting-edge science, researchers can stay ahead of emerging infectious threats and bolster population immunity.

Behavioural nudges and incentives may be employed to motivate vaccine uptake and foster a sense of collective responsibility towards achieving herd immunity. Strategies like vaccine lotteries, rewards programs, and social recognition initiatives can encourage individuals to get vaccinated and contribute to the greater good of community protection. By tapping into human psychology and social dynamics, public health interventions can nudge behaviour towards pro-vaccination attitudes and practices.

The ongoing monitoring of immunity levels, vaccine effectiveness, and disease dynamics will be crucial for adapting herd immunity strategies to changing epidemiological landscapes. Surveillance systems, serosurveys, and mathematical modelling can offer insights into the dynamics of immunity within populations, guiding decision-making on vaccination policies, booster strategies, and containment measures. By remaining vigilant and responsive to emerging trends, stakeholders can sustain and enhance herd

immunity to safeguard public health in the long term.

Chapter 15: Conclusion and Recommendations

In conclusion, achieving herd immunity to combat infectious diseases such as COVID-19 is a complex and multifaceted challenge that requires a coordinated effort from individuals, communities, governments, and public health organisations. The concept of herd immunity relies on a significant portion of the population becoming immune to the pathogen, either through vaccination or previous infection, thereby reducing its ability to spread within the community. While herd immunity can provide a level of protection against infectious diseases, it is crucial to approach this strategy with caution and consideration of various factors to ensure its effectiveness and sustainability.

Moving forward, it is imperative to prioritize vaccination campaigns to increase immunity levels within the population and reduce the spread of infectious diseases. Adequate vaccine distribution, accessibility, and education are key factors in achieving herd immunity and preventing future outbreaks. Furthermore, public health initiatives should focus on addressing vaccine hesitancy and misinformation to build trust in the safety and efficacy of vaccines. Encouraging widespread vaccination uptake through targeted messaging and community engagement can help accelerate the progress towards herd immunity.

Additionally, continued surveillance and monitoring of vaccination coverage rates, infection rates, and emerging variants are essential for assessing the progress towards herd immunity and adapting public health strategies accordingly. Regular testing, contact tracing, and genomic sequencing can provide valuable insights into the dynamics of disease transmission and help identify potential gaps in immunity within the population. By staying informed and proactive in addressing evolving challenges, stakeholders can better position themselves to achieve and maintain herd immunity over the long term.

It is also important to recognize that achieving herd immunity is not a one-size-fits-all solution, as different communities and regions may face unique barriers and considerations in reaching optimal immunity levels. Tailoring strategies to address specific needs, such as reaching vulnerable populations, implementing targeted vaccination campaigns, and collaborating with local stakeholders, can help overcome obstacles and foster a more inclusive approach to building immunity within communities. Emphasising equity, accessibility, and inclusivity in vaccination efforts is crucial for ensuring that no one is left behind in the journey towards herd immunity.

Moreover, ongoing research and investment in vaccine development, novel therapeutics, and public health infrastructure are key priorities for strengthening global immunity and resilience against infectious diseases. Collaboration between governments, researchers, industry stakeholders, and international organisations is essential for advancing scientific knowledge, innovation, and preparedness for future health crises. By fostering a culture of collaboration and knowledge sharing, stakeholders can leverage collective expertise and resources to address complex health challenges and enhance global health security.

In conclusion, achieving herd immunity requires a comprehensive and concerted effort from all stakeholders to increase immunity levels within the population, reduce disease transmission, and protect public health. By prioritising vaccination, addressing vaccine hesitancy, investing in public health infrastructure, and promoting equitable access to healthcare services, societies can work towards building a resilient immune system that can effectively combat infectious diseases and promote overall well-being. While the road to herd immunity may present challenges, by remaining vigilant, adaptable, and united in our efforts, we can pave the way for a healthier and more secure future for generations to come.